GW01017934

As Little As Possible *Most* of the Time

A SIMPLE WAY OF EATING THAT WILL SATISFY YOU WHILE EATING HEALTHY, SMALLER PORTIONS!

JANE HAASE

authorHOUSE®

AuthorHouse™
1663 Liberty Drive, Suite 200
Bloomington, IN 47403
www.authorhouse.com
Phone: 1-800-839-8640

First published by AuthorHouse 3/14/2008

ISBN: 978-1-4343-5970-4 (sc)

Printed in the United States of America
Bloomington, Indiana

This book is printed on acid-free paper.

Dedication

I dedicate this book to my two beautiful daughters, Ashley and Megan. I wrote the book with them in mind. It is my desire for them to live a life filled with healthy choices, quality fitness, and happiness ALWAYS!

Table of Contents

Introduction

"As Little As Possible, Most Of The Time". One may think that this is a challenging way to eat. First of all, this is NOT a diet. It is a simple plan to follow without using fad diets or gimmicks to lose weight. It is a set of habits you can utilize to stay healthy, to keep your desired weight, OR to lose weight. It is a way of eating that you can sustain for the rest of your life. I chose the title because as little as possible, most of the time is the way I look at everything I eat. No, I don't eat like a mouse and become emaciated because I am starving. I do however pay attention to the portions I eat and to what I eat. In other words, smaller portions all the time and healthy choices ALWAYS. This is what it is all about. And, it is very simple to do. This concept allows me to eat just about everything I want without denying myself the things I love to eat. It allows me to eat chocolate everyday and to have those special yummy foods that I crave and enjoy. The end result, a lifetime of enjoyable eating.

With this common sense approach to food, you can utilize this way of eating whether you are trying to lose weight or you are trying to maintain your weight. You do not need to count calories any more. You do not need to step on the scale everyday. You do not have to deny yourself the foods that add enjoyment to your life. This eating plan calls for eating as little as possible whenever given the opportunity to eat. Whenever you have a meal, you have a portion of most everything and NO seconds. You can eat when you want, as long as your food choices are healthy ones that will help your body, not make it sick. Depending on whether you want to lose weight or maintain your weight, you can modify this healthy way of eating to suit you. By avoiding unhealthy, processed foods and concentrating on foods to nourish your body as well at eating smaller portions most of the time, you will be successful in your goal.

I came up with the idea for my book while I was out walking my dog one sunny Saturday morning. I thought about my 21 year old daughter, Ashley and my 17 year old daughter, Megan and I wrote the book with them in mind. I remembered back to my 21st birthday and what I used to eat. That was when I weighed 180 pounds at 5'10". I saw my daughters making the same mistakes I did. I saw them making bad eating choices without being aware of what they were doing and without being very healthy. Consequently, filling themselves with junk food and gaining/losing weight in that yo-yo cycle we are all aware of. I wanted to pass on to them some of my tips on how to lose a few pounds, to stay healthy, and to maintain their weight the rest of their lives.

When I was 21, I used to go to a fast food restaurant on my lunch break. I would order a pork tenderloin sandwich (a midwestern sandwich of a breaded, highly salted, deep-fried pork cutlet on a bun), a large order of fries, and a large cola. I would eat this way Monday through Friday. I would devour the entire lunch during my 30-minute break and then wonder why at 3:00p.m. I could hardly keep my eyes open. To top it off, earlier in the day I would have eaten two sprinkle donuts for breakfast and break. I had NO idea what I was doing to myself. All I knew is that is tasted delicious.

At age 25, after years of eating poorly, I weighed 185 pounds. I was tired and lethargic most of the time. I did absolutely NO exercise and felt down and depressed often. What I didn't realize is that my unhealthy diet and lack of exercise had everything to do with this. Then I discovered walking. I started taking a 30 minute walk everyday after work and low and behold, I started enjoying this. I began to feel more alive each day. I began to take more of an interest in my body. By walking, I started to tone up my leg muscles and firm up my bottom. The more I walked, the more turned on to it I became. I haven't stopped since. This short walk of 30 minutes a day and a few diet modifications allowed me to eat what I wanted and to maintain my weight, perhaps even lose a pound or two. The walking became my way of keeping in shape, at the same time it gave me a way to de-stress my life just a little bit.

My eating habits did not change much until I was pregnant with my first daughter at age 28. I started becoming more aware of the importance of vitamins and minerals in my diet because of my pregnancy. I added fruits and vegetables to my diet a few times a week (yes, I said a few times a week). I increased my protein intake because I realized this was important for the baby I was carrying. I drank milk, but chocolate milk it was. My habit of eating everything I wanted all the time shifted to eating a more balanced, nutritious diet. And, I kept walking. I started to walk longer than 30 minutes and at a quicker pace up until the time I gave birth. I gained 25 pounds during pregnancy and gave birth to a healthy baby girl.

After Ashley was born, I became very active taking care of her. I was so busy that I lost the 25 pounds I gained during my pregnancy. I continued my love of walking and included 30+ minutes of walking a day with baby in stroller or front carrier. My diet remained better than in my younger years, but I also developed some bad eating habits once again. I would get so exhausted at times that I started to binge eat for quick energy. I followed this by not eating anything for 12-24 hours. My binge eating consisted of going to the grocery store and buying pastries and ice cream. Then, I would go home and devour most of it in one sitting. Then because of guilt, I would not eat for a while and skip meals and nutritious food. My life had changed dramatically with a new baby and whether I liked it or not, I was forced to become a mother and provider for someone other than me, namely Ashley. I loved my daughter dearly, but my life was no longer what it used to be. So, I ate to make myself feel better. Then I would go hungry to compensate for overeating. You might call this anorexic, but I never did. I never recognized this in myself and 20 years ago, this disease was not spoken of much. I just did it because it made me feel good. The only good thing about this eating pattern was that I continued to walk and to add different exercises to my life to compensate for overeating.

My second daughter was born 4 years later. After her birth and having two small children at home, there was no way I could keep up with my binge eating. Why? Because it would totally exhaust me and I now needed my energy to raise a family. I started to improve my diet slightly and to lose weight. I also added swimming laps as a form of exercise to make myself feel better. I would swim freestyle laps for 30 minutes, 5 times a week in addition to walking. Swimming to me is a wonderful form of exercise because I can do it by myself (which I like) and it is absolutely invigorating. There is something about being in the water that is cleansing and rejuvenating. The more I swam, the stronger and slimmer I got. I soon weighed 145 pounds. I started reading more and more about fruits and vegetables, proteins, carbohydrates, fats, sugars, and the good and bad in these foods and what they can do to help or break down your body. I read everything I could on nutrition and became very knowledgeable about diet. I started realizing that everything I put in my body would either make it better or make it sick.

This is when I started eating as little as possible, most of the time. And once again, I want you to realize that I do NOT eat like a bird and act anorexic. But I do become more aware of what I am putting into my body. I look at everything I eat and I do not take large helpings of anything like I used to do in the past. Instead, I choose smaller portions whenever possible and healthy choices ALWAYS. It has become my way of life and is a common sense approach to eating. If I am trying to lose weight and relied on counting calories, I would eat between 1500 and 1800 calories per day and watch closely what I eat. If I am trying to maintain my weight, I have many more options and can add more foods that I enjoy. However, my focus is not on counting calories, but rather on eating healthy. I have learned some tricks about eating that help me stay about the same weight and give me more energy. It is my desire now to stay healthy and maintain the same weight. I also knew that if I wanted to live a long life, I needed to feed my body well in addition to exercising. I realized that my heart is a muscle also and it was up to me to keep it in shape.

I knew then that one of the most important things that I wanted to do for myself was to continue walking OR do some form of exercise everyday. To me walking was the easiest to fit into my everyday life. I realized how important walking was to me and that there was NO excuse not to do this simple exercise called walking everyday. I knew I could fit 30 minutes into my daily life to take a walk. I haven't stopped since. I have walked in 100 degree weather and I have walked in minus 1 degree weather while visiting Iowa, the state where I was born and raised. I walk in the rain with an umbrella or hooded jacket. I walk fast or I walk leisurely depending on how I feel and who I am with. Sometimes I jog too, depending on how my knees feel. Sometimes I walk more than 30 minutes and that is certainly to my advantage. It doesn't take special clothing or equipment, just good shoes. I have established a route around my neighborhood that takes 30 minutes to walk. I also have several other places that I like to walk that take longer. It is especially invigorating for me to walk in the morning. Sometimes I walk right away when I get home from work. I love to walk the dogs in my family and they of course love it too. When I come back from a walk, I always feel better mentally. If the weather is inclement, I sometimes go to the shopping mall and walk inside. I usually figure out most of my life's problems by the time I am done taking my walk. No seriously, it is a great way to clear the mind of extra clutter.

If for some reason I can't walk on a particular day, I do anything else I can think of that is active. I have a yoga and an aerobic DVD that I put on in my living room and exercise with. I have a set of 5 pound weights that I work out with for my arms. I belong to a fitness club that I go to occasionally and walk/run on the treadmill for 30 minutes. I dance to some upbeat music. The most important thing is that 30 minutes a day, I become active and increase my heart rate. If I need to lose weight, the more of these activities I do.

In addition to the exercise, I am constantly aware of what I am feeding my body. I know everything I put in my mouth can make a difference. Healthy, fresh food of course is the best. I know the importance of fruits and vegetables and what they can do to repair and help my insides stay healthy. I know I must have some protein daily to stay alert. I know that fat is O.K. to eat, but in reduced portions. I know carbohydrates give me quick energy, but too much of them can be harmful. And I also know that I need chocolate every day and special treats in my life to make it more enjoyable. When I go to my grave, I want to say that I have enjoyed myself along the way! I eat 3 pieces of chocolate each day and that takes care of my chocolate craving. I eat special higher calorie treats once a week because I know that if I deny myself these foods all the time, I will fail. Of course it still takes "will power", but if you think of how you are helping your body, the will power to eat properly will come easier. This habit of eating works for me!

I am 53 years old now and have not fluctuated 5 pounds over or below my weight of 145 pounds for many years. If I gain 5 pounds in the winter, that is O.K. with me. I usually lose it back in the spring and summer. If I start to gain more than 5 pounds, that is when I put the brakes on and get myself back on track. If my clothes start to feel too tight, then I know I need to concentrate on healthy eating habits and make sure I am getting the proper 30 minutes of exercise a day. I don't deprive myself of things I like to eat. Rather I allow myself to eat these things with moderation. MODERATION is the key word here. There is so much food in this world to eat, why not enjoy it while you are alive to do so. But with MODERATION. It is very simple. No diet. Just sensible eating combined with some exercise every day.

This book is written in general for women of all ages. However, men should be able to follow this set of eating habits also. Men ALSO need to pay attention to the portions they eat. They will be able to eat more food than what I have outlined in my book because in general, they are bigger than women. NO SECONDS is a big issue for men. Remember your portions and don't eat until you are bloated. Exercise is also important to men. The 30 minute walk a day is a nice activity to do with your mate or significant other. You will discover that you may communicate differently and perhaps more calmly while on a walk.

I hope you will enjoy my book. It is truly a common sense way to eat and to maintain your weight happily. I have broken the book down into chapters that I found to be the most beneficial. If you need to lose weight first, then really concentrate on adding more fruits and vegetables to your diet and smaller portions. And, stay active. WALK, WALK, WALK! It is so simple to do. Then, maintain with happiness. Focus on your health, not on your weight. You will be successful!

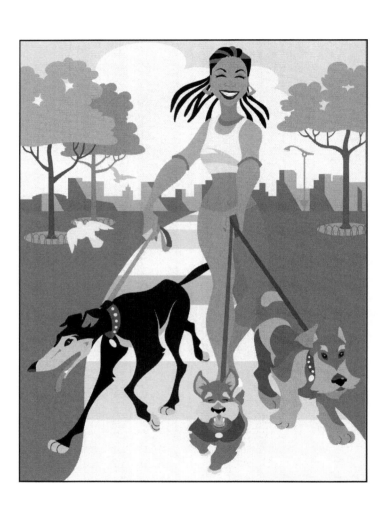

CHAPTER 1

Exercise

As I mentioned before, the best gift you can give to your health is to walk at least 30 minutes everyday. There is NO excuse why you can't fit that into each and every day. Here are some other tips that I found beneficial to add to my exercise regime:

+ walk briskly or as fast as possible, but don't overdo it because you want to enjoy yourself
+ wear good shoes with a good arch support
+ get a dog to walk, borrow your neighbor's dog (unless of course you have your own dog), take it for a walk, the dog will love you
+ whenever you are bored, take a walk
+ use the inside of a shopping mall if the weather is unpleasant
+ walking will ALWAYS make you feel better
+ walking makes you feel rejuvenated and gives you motivation
+ you can substitute other exercise if you want, but remember at least 30 minutes a day i.e.; swimming,

fitness club, biking, running, tennis, dancing, yoga, weights

+ raking and sweeping outside in your yard is a great exercise
+ to complement the walking and to build up your arm muscles, use 3-5 pound weights (at a different time than your walk) to build up your arm muscles, walking will take care of strengthening your leg muscles and keep your fanny firm
+ buy a "Jock Jams" CD and put it on and dance to it (you won't be able to sit down when you hear the music)
+ find an aerobics class, yoga, or Jazzercise class to attend
+ Richard Simmons has a great work out tape called "Disco Sweat", obtain a copy of that if you can, it is 40 minutes of great exercise
+ drink water before you exercise and after
+ remember, you must USE your muscles or they will shrink up into little puff balls, this includes your heart muscle too

If you want to combine walking and jogging together to obtain a more cardiovascular workout once in a while, try this easy formula:

Walk 2 minutes, jog 10 minutes at an easy pace, jog faster for 2 minutes, walk briskly for 2 minutes, jog for 10 minutes, walk 2 minutes briskly to cool down, walk slower the last 2 minutes. Total time=30 minutes. If you want to jog for the entire 30 minutes, start out with this easy pattern and eventually you will be able to jog the entire ½ hour.

CHAPTER 2

Fruits & Vegetables

You have heard it before, now you will hear it again. EAT your veggies. They say to eat 6 servings of fruit daily and 6 servings of vegetables daily, but my goal is to have 6 servings combined in a day. Any more than that is of course good for you, so I try to eat as many as possible. Every time I eat a fruit or veggie, I remind myself that I am making my body so much healthier. This gives me the motivation to keep it up. Take a glance at my tips!

+ never eat canned fruits and vegetables, only fresh
+ eat your colors, try to eat fruits and veggies in a variety of colors which will give you different vitamins and minerals from each
+ don't worry too much about the serving size, just make sure you get a minimum of 6 servings a day (hopefully more)
+ make fruit salads by mixing different kinds of fruits together...it is delicious
+ the less candy and sugar you eat, the sweeter the fruit will taste, trust me, it's true

- make a low-cal veggie dip to dip your broccoli and carrots in (recipe to follow), but don't overdo the dipping
- always have cup up veggies in your refrigerator for snacking
- try some new veggies you've never tried before, try new veggie recipes
- sometimes I take 3 large pieces of broccoli and stuff it in my mouth and eat it because I know what a fantastic vegetable it is for my body
- microwave frozen vegetables, try sprinkling parmesan cheese on them
- in my opinion, a banana is as close to a perfect food as possible, loaded with nutrition
- try to eat some tomato everyday, it too is loaded with nutrition
- soy beans have great vegetable protein and fiber in them
- potatoes are O.K. in moderation, the have great potassium in them
- never eat iceberg lettuce, no nutrition, the darker the lettuce the more vitamins
- every time you eat fruits or veggies, give yourself a pat on the back for staying healthy
- try eating salsa as a salad dressing, it is low cal, good for you, and tasty
- avoid eating heavy, creamy salad dressings, chose an oil based dressing instead

Delicious Dill Dip

16 oz. container of fat free sour cream
16 oz. of fat free mayonnaise
2 T. dill weed
2 T. onion flakes
1 t. seasoned salt

Mix all ingredients together. Let sit in refrigerator
for 24 hrs. Eat. ENJOY! It is great for veggies

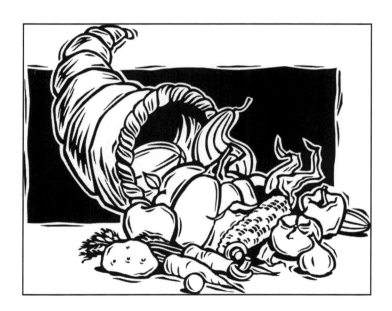

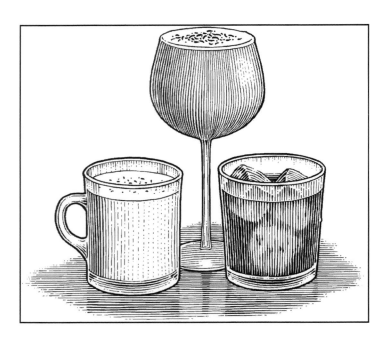

CHAPTER 3

Beverages

What you drink can add up to a lot of wasted calories. By that I mean very little nutritional value, lots of sugar. I prefer to eat my calories rather than drink them!

+ eat an apple or an orange rather than drinking orange juice or apple juice, it is more filling and has the added fiber to go along with it
+ limit yourself to 1 diet cola a day, anymore could increase your caffeine intake which in turn will make you more hungry
+ have coffee in the morning, decaf in the afternoon
+ drink at least 2 cups of milk a day, either by the glass or on your cereal, I like 2%, but 1% or skim is better if you are trying to lose weight
+ milk is excellent and makes your teeth white and bones stronger
+ with your milk, I suggest taking a vitamin D/with calcium tablet to help your bones, calcium is absorbed better along with the vitamin D

- use Crystal Light to drink if you require something sweet in the afternoon
- no Starbucks fancy Frappuccinos if you are trying to lose pounds, they can have as much as 500 calories in them
- if you like to go to coffee shops, order plain coffee with milk and a sweetener if you must, it should taste sweet enough to take care of that sweet tooth
- hot chocolate is a wasted drink, unless of course you make it with milk
- no fancy Hawaiian tropical alcoholic drinks (unless of course you are in Hawaii on vacation), they are loaded with sugar
- if you like to party, drink lite beer, wine, or mixed drinks made with alcohol and club soda, tonic, or diet cola
- put lots of ice in your alcoholic drink and make that drink last a long time
- and of course, drink plenty of that good stuff called water everyday

One of my favorite snacks is this nutritional smoothie that I make in my blender. It is very good for you because it is high in calcium and delicious. Try it!

1 ripe banana
1 T. dry milk powder
1 cup low fat yogurt
3 ice cubes
½ cup skim milk
½ t. vanilla

Blend together in a blender. Enjoy!

CHAPTER 4

Pastries And Sweets

Pastries are my weakness. I love baked goods like cinnamon rolls, cookies, cakes, pies, and best of all doughnuts! I know that if I choose to eat a doughnut, I will feel lethargic and tired a couple of hours later. This is because of the fat and sugar content in the doughnut. So if I have one, I choose the time to eat one wisely. If you are trying to lose weight, the fewer pastries you should eat until you are trying to maintain your weight. Then you may be able to add a few more. Cakes and cupcakes are a fact of life. They will always be around. Don't deny yourself these. Just remember, as little as possible most of the time. Some other ideas to keep in mind:

+ if you crave a doughnut, have ONE occasionally, it won't kill you
+ if possible, have a glass of milk with your doughnut as it will add the needed protein to keep your energy up and you will not feel so tired later in the day

- even though you may think you are doing yourself a favor by eating a muffin, they can be loaded with fat and have more calories than a doughnut
- if you must have a muffin, eat ½ now and ½ tomorrow
- try not to eat an entire bagel, just ½ with a little cream cheese or jelly
- if you want to have a whole bagel, take the middle, doughy part out and just eat the outside, less constipating
- if someone brings a birthday cake to work or school, take only ONE piece and make it a small one, eat it all (including the frosting if you must), maybe exercise a little bit more later in the day or eat a little less
- PANCAKES get a BAD RAP! Pancakes are O.K. if you eat them with NO butter and light syrup. I like to make an individual pancake (or waffle) using ½ cup low fat bisquick, one egg, one egg white, and milk for consistency, the extra egg white is for added protein, this usually takes care of my pancake craving
- COOKIES....the most difficult to say NO to for some of us....try not to keep them in the house if you can't resist the urge, don't eat more than 3 at a time, preferably with milk, if you feel like eating more, take a walk instead
- when eating pie, try not to eat the crust if you are trying to lose, if you are maintaining and the crust is HOMEMADE, go ahead and enjoy, store bought crust isn't worth it!
- NO sweet rolls, they are nothing but bad
- a few small candies everyday is O.K. like chocolate kisses (3 have only 100 calories), candy corn, junior

mints, jelly beans, orange slices…..no more than 3-8 (depending on the candy), once again, don't keep it in the house if you can't stop yourself, dark chocolate has been proven to be the best for you, I try never to have a large candy bar, rather a small one if I am maintaining, chew gum instead!

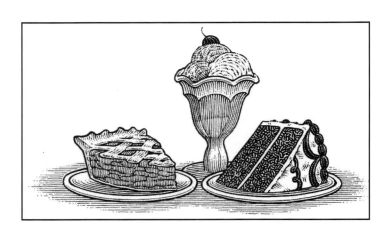

CHAPTER 5

Special Treats

Rewarding yourself with a special treat occasionally is a nice thing to do. If I exercise extra long or work extra hard around the house, I usually give myself something I really enjoy to eat. Once again, this depends on whether you are maintaining or losing weight. Usually once a week I go buy myself something I really enjoy like a McDonald's McFlurry, a piece of pie, a Jamba Juice, a Wendy's frosty, a bacon cheeseburger, an order of onion rings, etc. Denying these things would not be fun and may set you up for failure. By doing this just occasionally, it gives you something to look forward to. Most diets are too rigid and very restrictive about treats. You have a better chance of being successful if you allow yourself these special goodies. What is your favorite treat?

Mine is ice cream, but.....

+ never keep ice cream in your freezer at home if you are tempted to eat the entire carton, if you want it go buy it for your special treat

- McDonald's ice cream cones and sundaes are very small, tasty, and cheap
- do not buy food at the movies, resist the urge and save the $$$
- as much as possible, try to avoid white flour products and white sugar products
- cut out extremely fatty treats as they will make you tired, rather make a different choice
- a Pina Colada or a Long Island Iced Tea with a few appetizers would be a treat
- if you have a craving for a fast food burger, go ahead and get one, save the french fries or onion rings for next time
- when eating chips, take a portion from the bag and put them in a bowl, eat only that amount and do not eat directly from the bag
- if you go to an ice cream parlor and you are trying to lose weight, order a kid's scoop....an hour later you won't have missed that extra portion of ice cream
- if you go to a baseball or football game, buy peanuts and enjoy eating them during the game, they will take a while to eat......try to avoid garlic fries
- enjoy your special treat, eat it slowly and savor it
- if you do find yourself eating more than you should have, add a little bit more exercise that day or eat less the following meal

Once again, if you have reached your desired weight and want to maintain, you can experiment with these special treats and add more to your diet. If you are trying to lose weight and "blow it" one day, don't be too hard on yourself. This happens to all of us. Try to get back on track. If you have a craving for some junk food, try waiting for 10 minutes and the craving will usually go away. Just remember that tomorrow is another day and you can start eating healthy once again!

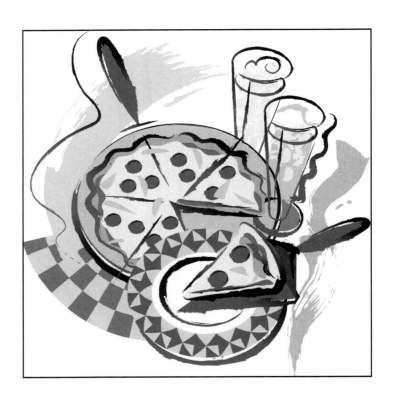

CHAPTER 6

Going Out To Eat

Going out to eat is a fact of life and it is FUN! I try to limit my restaurant visits as I am always tempted to overeat. Plus, you save money by staying home. Remember to eat slowly. Your body does not tell you that you are full until 20 minutes later. On a scale of 1-10 with 10 being extremely full and uncomfortable, try to remain at a 5 so that you are satisfied, but not stuffed. There are other ways to make wise choices and enjoy......

- always order something on the menu that doesn't appear TOO large
- if you want a hamburger, go ahead and order it, if possible blot off some of the extra fat on the burger with a napkin (I have been known to put my napkin around the burger and squeeze the fat out)
- to your burger only add tomato, lettuce, onions, mustard, and ketchup if you are trying to lose, you can add a little mayo and cheese if you are maintaining
- take off the bun if you have already had too many carbohydrates that day

- try to avoid ordering french fries, instead steal 5-6 off you husband or child's plate....try not to eat an entire order as they are usually quite large
- salads are good, but avoid the heavy dressings, order on the side if you must
- limit croutons on your salad to 5-6
- grilled chicken sandwiches are a good choice
- if you get a huge meal at a restaurant, take ½ home for your next meal, it will taste even better as a leftover
- try to eat your largest meal at lunchtime, not dinner
- for breakfast at a restaurant, order a senior breakfast: 2 eggs, 2 sausages, and whole wheat toast, skip the hash browns
- pancakes are O.K., but only with light syrup and no butter
- only eat 1 large piece of pizza or 2 small pieces
- Subway has great sandwiches which include meat, lots of veggies, and are low-cal...just ask Jared
- when ordering a sandwich at a deli, avoid heaving dressings, instead use mustard
- bean and cheese burritos are usually good for you because of the protein and fiber
- super burritos have a lot of calories because of the sour cream and guacamole, if you have one, try to eat ½ today and ½ tomorrow
- if you go to a buffet restaurant, eat ONLY the things you like the most and skip the rest....use your will power
- at buffet lines, I usually take a very small salad (if any) because I can eat salads at home, rather I eat a lot of meat and vegetables, small portions of potatoes, pasta dishes, and breads

- one dessert at a buffet........use your will power!
- Chinese food is full of fat and salt, try to have it only occasionally
- I usually eat all my airplane meals because I am hungry, bored, and stressed...that is just the way it is! (airline food always tastes good to me...even if it is just peanuts!)

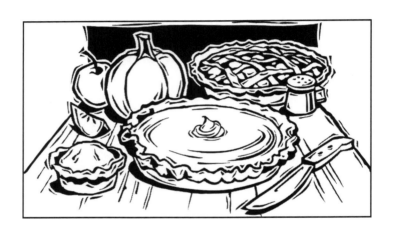

CHAPTER 7

Holidays

Around the holiday time, it is especially hard to stay "on track" with eating. Most of us celebrate Thanksgiving and have the privilege of eating a meal with all the trimmings. We usually all go to one or more Christmas parties which always include food and beverages. If you can simply stay at your weight during these times, you are doing great. Try not to overeat so that you have to make a New Year's resolution to go on a diet and then fail by February 1st. Stick with eating as little as possible most of the time and you should do fine. Always prepare yourself before you go to these parties and eat something before you go so you are not starving. If you do overindulge, the next day you can exercise a little bit more and start eating properly again. Remember that scale of 1-10….try to keep it at a 5 as far as feeling full. Don't beat up on yourself for slipping once in a while. Enjoy the holidays with all its many splendors and……

- make socializing with people more important than snacking
- stand away from the food table, you will be less tempted to overindulge
- limit your alcoholic consumption, make your drinks last a long time, add ice
- eat healthy foods before you go
- volunteer to bring something that you know you will be able to eat
- at Thanksgiving, eat a lot of turkey (protein), vegetables, and salad; take a small portion of mashed potatoes, gravy, stuffing, roll, and pumpkin pie. You may not lose a pound that day and you may even gain a pound however, you will have enjoyed yourself, get back on track the day after
- give away some of your leftovers
- when you go to a Christmas party, take only the appetizers that you really enjoy and skip the rest, later that evening you'll be glad you did
- if there are many Christmas cookies at a party, only take 1-3 cookies that you REALLY, REALLY like, savor each one, you don't need any more than that
- enjoy baking Christmas cookies at home, but try to resist the urge to eat them all, give some to your neighbors or co-workers
- don't quit walking during the holidays, it is especially important at this time to continue your fitness
- remember to use your will power, remind yourself to eat healthy first and eat as little as possible of the wrong foods

CHAPTER 8

Breakfast, Lunch, Dinner, & Snacks

It is important to eat three meals each day. Most health experts agree that skipping breakfast is a no no. I agree with this. The energy you derive from eating breakfast will help you stay on track with eating during the day. It will also help you remain more alert for your work day and to have more energy. My day usually includes:

+ Breakfast
+ Snack
+ Lunch
+ Snack
+ Dinner
+ Snack

I never let myself get hungry because I hate the feeling of an empty stomach. There are always good choices to make if you need to snack. If you are trying to lose weight, then of course you must be careful about snacking. You will also need to choose lighter snacks and meals throughout the day until you reach your desired weight. If you are trying to maintain your weight, you can experiment with different kinds of snacks and see what works for you. Some people can eat and snack more than others. You will need to determine what it takes to keep you on track. And of course, the more exercise you add to your day, the better. If you are trying to lose weight, the added exercise will help you lose faster. If you are trying to maintain, the added exercise will allow you to eat more that day. The more muscles you have, the more calories you will burn even at a resting state. So building stronger, firmer muscles is to your advantage. And remember, the minimum amount of fitness a day is 30 minutes of walking…..that is it, no more if you don't want to.

Figure out when your weakest part of the day is for snacking. Have a game plan of what you might do to get through this time. If you start overeating, get out of the house for a while. Change your surroundings. In 5 or 10 minutes the urge will pass and you will not have filled yourself up with loaded snacks. Always have veggies in the refrigerator. Remember that each time you put these in your mouth, you are becoming healthier and stronger, not to mention they fill your stomach and are good for your digestive system. Drinking water is also important at this time. I like to have a cup of instant decaffeinated coffee in the afternoon with a little milk and artificial sweetener. This along with a snack, helps me get through that 4:00p.m. doldrums. Try to limit your carbohydrates during this time, rather concentrate on eating more proteins. Eating enough protein is VERY important to keep you alert, to keep your muscles strong, and to give you energy. Milk is an excellent source of protein. Other foods you might try at this time would be yogurt, eggs, soy beans, nuts, protein bar, or cheese. Think healthy, healthy, healthy, not diet, diet, diet. The fact that you may increase your life expectancy by eating healthy SHOULD give you more incentive to eat well. I have included a sample of meals and snacks that I eat in a day:

Breakfast

+ a bowl of high fiber cereal with milk and ½ banana
+ one container of low fat yogurt with fresh berries, glass of milk
+ 1 scrambled egg with 1 piece of whole wheat toast, glass of milk
+ 1 individual pancake with light syrup (see recipe in the pastry section)
+ one piece of whole wheat toast with peanut butter, glass of milk
+ oatmeal with milk, one serving of fruit
+ cream of wheat (it is high in iron), milk to drink

I have found that oatmeal keeps me the fullest for the longest. Try to eat the oatmeal that takes 5 minutes to cook, not the one-minute quick oats. The old-fashioned type of oatmeal has more fiber in it and is better for combating cholesterol. If you have a big test or presentation to give that morning, make it a 2-egg breakfast with toast. The protein in the eggs will help you stay alert and more energetic longer throughout the morning.

Snack (midmorning)

+ one bowl of fresh mixed fruit
+ one handful of almonds or walnuts (about 1 oz. or 8-10 nuts)
+ one container of low fat yogurt
+ one banana and 3-4 nuts
+ one breakfast bar
+ one hard boiled egg
+ 3-4 rice crackers
+ a cheese stick and apple slices

You get the idea, small portions most of the time, but enough to keep you from feeling hungry.

Lunch

+ a sandwich made with 1 piece of whole wheat bread, slice of cheese, 3-4 slices of meat, 6-8 tortilla chips, one piece of fruit, milk or diet drink
+ 1 piece of whole wheat bread with peanut butter and jelly, 6-8 potato chips, one cookie, water or diet drink
+ one bean and cheese burrito (add rice to give it more protein)
+ one Subway roast beef or turkey sandwich with drink
+ ½ of the left over meal you ordered at the restaurant last night
+ salad with tuna, tomatoes, fresh vegetables, and light Italian dressing
+ one medium to large piece of pizza, drink
+ 1 Lean Cuisine microwavable meal and milk
+ grilled cheese sandwich made with whole wheat bread, milk to drink

Be creative with what you eat. Remember, the most important thing is the portion size. You can have what you want with moderation. Don't eat 20-30 chips, but rather have a smaller portion. Have pizza, but not the entire pizza!

Snack (mid-afternoon)

- bowl of mixed fruit
- soy nuts, ½ cup, they are great for the symptoms of menopause
- yogurt with fruit
- nuts (almonds, walnuts, or mixed nuts) 1 oz.
- 2 small cookies with a cup of decaf
- 6-8 wheat thins with melted cheese
- popcorn (low or no butter)
- an ice cream cone from McDonald's
- veggies with dill dip
- toasted pita bread with peanut butter or cheese
- rye-crisp with a little cream cheese
- apple slices with cheese
- vegetable soup (homemade is better, canned is O.K.)

One of my favorite snacks to have in the refrigerator is a mixture of jello and cool whip layered together to look like a fancy dessert. You can use sugar free jello and fat free cool whip if you like. The texture is very satisfying and it is simple, light, and delicious.

Afternoon time would be a perfect time to get out of the house and take a walk, go to the grocery store, do some gardening, take a cat nap, anything to take you out of your surroundings that make you want to overeat. Once again, if you want to lose weight, lighter snacks. To maintain your weight, a little bit more.

Dinner

+ meat and salad, hot vegetables (grill your meat if possible), meat should be about the size of the palm of your hand
+ if you like to make casseroles for your family, eat a small portion with a side of hot veggies or salad
+ soup and salad
+ try to avoid making boxed pasta, rice, or potato dishes...full of salt, preservatives, and not much nutrition
+ try whole wheat pasta (about 1 cup) with Italian dressing or sprinkled with parmesan cheese
+ fish is great 2-3 times a week, try to avoid red meat as much as possible
+ buy yourself a cookbook that emphasizes cooking light
+ baked potatoes are O.K., try to have just a little bit of butter, nothing else
+ steamed vegetables are great, try sprinkling them with Molly McButter
+ Lean Cuisine meals are quick and easy if you are alone
+ scrambled eggs and toast is good too if you have nothing else
+ DO NOT have desserts in the house if you have trouble staying away from them...if you want something, go out and get it

One of my favorite quick easy meals to fix for myself and my family are chicken tortilla roll-ups. They are delicious and easy. Try them!

4-8" whole wheat tortillas
1 lb. cooked chicken or turkey, cut up
½ can refried beans
2 oz. sliced red onion
2 oz. shredded lettuce
4 tsp. cilantro

Mix all the ingredients together in a bowl, spread on tortillas and roll up. Serve hot or cold. You can spread the tortillas with humus or salsa before topping with the mixture to add moisture. This meal is very high in protein and can be used at lunch or dinner.

Try not to eat after 8:00p.m. Brush and floss your teeth at that time so you will be less tempted to eat again. My favorite evening snack is a glass of milk. It fills me up and helps me sleep well. I also like string cheese or yogurt in the evening. It is VERY important not to go to bed after eating a huge meal. Try to make your biggest meal at lunch, not dinner. If you overeat in the evening, try to take a walk the next morning and eat a lighter breakfast. Experiment with your evening snack and see what works best for you. I have to mention insomnia at this point. If you are hungry, you will not sleep well. So, avoid going to bed hungry. You will most likely wake up in the middle of the night and raid the refrigerator. Some other techniques I use to help me get to sleep are:

- unclench your fists and relax both hands, it will help you relax
- when you first get into bed, do 1-2 minutes of deep breathing while laying flat on your back (breath in through your nose and out through your mouth..... slowly)
- turn the T.V. off, it is a stimulant
- visualize a calm, peaceful moment of your life
- if you can't sleep, get out of bed for 10-15 minutes, then come back and try again
- take a warm bath before bed
- drink warm milk before bed
- lay on your back on the floor with your legs against the wall facing straight up (so your body is at a right angle), lay that way for 10-15 minutes, a great yoga posture which stimulates circulation
- listen to soft music or nature sounds
- give closure to the day remembering the nice things that happened to you

CHAPTER 9

Care What You Look (And Feel) Like

The most important gift you can give yourself is to care who you are and what you look like. Never get too old or too lazy to let this go by the wayside. If you feel good about yourself, you will retain great motivation to stay healthy and at a good weight. I feel it is important to do these things on a regular basis:

+ put on make-up every day, even if it is just blush on the cheeks or color on your lips, it will make you feel brighter
+ wear jewelry like earrings, a necklace, a watch, anything to add sparkle to your appearance
+ shower everyday, fix your hair
+ dress youthful and with taste, don't wear sweats all the time
+ wear perfume
+ buy yourself one thing every month that will help you look and feel better

- stand up straight and tall
- don't smoke, it adds wrinkles to your face and ages you quickly
- brush and floss your teeth daily, several times a day
- don't stand on the scale every morning, rather maintain your weight by how your clothes fit
- wash your hands often, especially when you come home from shopping
- garden or rake outside, it is great for the soul
- protect your back every time you pick something up from the ground, bend your knees and stick out your butt
- be loving to someone everyday
- every night before you go to bed, think of one nice thing you did for someone that day
- if you get off track one day with your eating plan, notice how awful you feel (physically) and get right back at being healthy the next day
- if you are feeling down, eat some protein or carbohydrates for energy, carbs also release serotonin to your brain
- if you feel depressed, take a walk
- 20 minute cat naps can recharge you
- play with a cat or dog if you can, it can reduce stress
- try not to let other's problems become yours, give them the opportunity to learn and figure it out by themselves
- if you feel strongly about a certain issue, trying softening up about it and it will reduce the amount of stress that goes along with that issue
- look for the beauty in little things

- as the old saying goes, "Don't make a mountain out of a molehill"
- if you are having a miserable day, remind yourself that tomorrow you will have a fresh start and feel better......and you usually do

Start the day with OPTIMISM
Live the day with COMPASSION
End the day with LOVE

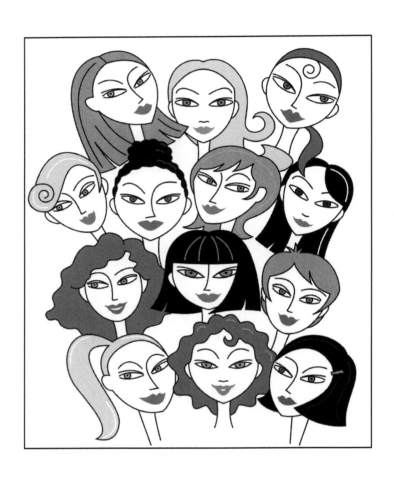

CHAPTER 10

Eat For Your Health

It is important that you remind yourself every day of how healthy you have become. Give yourself a pat on the back for eating fresh vitamins and minerals and not so much junk. Put foods in your mouth that will improve your body. You will no longer be eating to lose weight, but rather eating to stay healthy. If you eat healthier, you will lose weight or maintain your weight much easier. If you eat to be healthy, you will become a happier person. Your diet can bring you down or build you up. You have that choice. Use your will power and remind yourself of some of these things:

+ carrots have vitamin-A and beta-carotene in them which is important to vision
+ tomatoes contain lycopene which can reduce cancer risks
+ broccoli is a super food and helps guard against all kinds of cancer
+ leafy, dark green vegetables have high levels of vitamin A, phosphorous, iron, potassium, and calcium

49

- fruits are high in antioxidants which help neutralize toxins in our body
- fruits have a high amount of vitamin C to help you from getting sick
- whole grain breads and pasta add excellent fiber to your diet as well as vitamin B
- egg yolks are an important source of vitamin B-6 and B-12
- soy beans are the only vegetable that is a complete protein
- fats from whole foods are essential to our body and help us to absorb vitamins
- almonds contain serotonin which is a calming hormone, they can also reduce the LDL (bad cholesterol) in your body and raise the HDL (good cholesterol)
- omega-3, the "good fat" helps your memory and improves your brain function
- chocolate (especially dark) can trigger the release of endorphins in your body which will make you feel happier
- walking helps you maintain your balance, mobility, manage your weight, reduce stress, guard against heart disease, keep your bones strong, etc. etc. etc...need I say more
- too much sugar can increase the amount of insulin in your body and can cause diabetes
- red meats are very hard for your body to digest
- too many soft drinks can ruin your teeth

CHAPTER 11

Food Additives

Since it has been my goal to become a healthier eater, I feel that it is important to mention food additives. I want my girls to know that what they put in their mouth, even though they think it is very healthy, may have added chemicals that could increase their risk of disease. It is a fact that in the United States, as well as in other countries which we import our foods from, chemicals are added to food. They are used to enhance taste, improve appearance, and to preserve the quality of the food. I believe that the increase in cancer has a lot to do with the environment and the foods we eat. Even if you think you are eating a healthy piece of fruit, most of the time it has been treated with a pesticide to keep it fresh and to keep the bugs off. Organic foods are a good choice to consume because they are free of pesticides and additives. Many scientists are searching for preservatives from natural products, however they have a long way to go. I am trying to include more organic foods in my diet and it is my hope that my children will become more aware of the food they eat as they get older. Below I have mentioned just a few:

- MSG (monosodium glutamate) used in Chinese food, meat, poultry, seafood, and vegetables, can cause cancer and asthmatic reactions
- trans fat, found in crackers, cookies, margarine, can raise the LDL (bad cholesterol) and lower HDL (good cholesterol)
- artificial colorings such as yellow #6, blue #3, green #3, and red #3, found in candy, soda, gelatin, and more, can cause hyperactivity, thyroid problems, and allergic reactions
- sodium nitrite found in processed meats like bacon, ham, hot dogs, and lunchmeats, used to stop bacteria and produce the pink color, can cause cancer
- rBGH found in milk and milk products, dairy farmers inject their cows with it to improve milk production, can cause cancer
- pesticides used on fruit, farmers spray their produce with chemical fertilizers to keep insects and weeds at bay
- sulfites, used to preserve color and crispness, used with raisins and dried fruits, can trigger an asthmatic reaction, found also in some wines
- high-fructose corn syrup, found in frozen foods, sweets, breads, ketchup, and more, can increase your chance of diabetes and heart disease

I have just touched on a few food additives in which we should all try to avoid. This is a process I am just starting to discover. I am guilty of not eating the "best" foods all the time. However, it is my goal to eat more organic foods as well as to continue to read the labels on food products to see exactly what they contain. The sooner we all start doing this, the better chance we have of living a healthier life.

CHAPTER 12

Enjoy The Rest Of Your Life

There are two ideas to keep in mind after finishing this book. Aim for fitness and build a healthy diet. It is so simple. To me, the best form of fitness is that daily walk. How easy is that! Once you get in the routine of walking, you won't be able to do without it. I can't emphasize this enough. Build walking into your schedule so that walking becomes a priority in your life. It only takes ½ hour. Enjoy the outdoors while you walk. It is therapeutic to get yourself out of the house. Secondly, eat to keep your body healthy and functioning well. That is what food is for….to keep our engines running smoothly. Make those healthy choices instead of bad ones. Get motivated into eating correctly and notice how much better you will feel. Pay attention to the food pyramid. Eat fewer fats, oils, and sweets…..some milk, yogurt, and cheese as well as protein, nuts, eggs, and large portions of vegetables, fruits, and whole grains whenever possible. If you want to add a piece or two of chocolate into your diet every day, that is O.K. as long as you stay on track. Enjoy your special foods once a week. This should help you enjoy yourself along the way. Your will power will become stronger and stronger once you experience the results. Most likely you will feel better about yourself for choosing to be healthy. Choose also to be happy. Enjoy the small moments in life that make you smile. Don't get caught up in negativism. A negative attitude can ultimately make you sick. Look at everything as if it were happening for a reason. Believe in a higher power. Life is a pretty remarkable event. And once again, as little as possible MOST of the time. Watch your portions. Don't eat as if it were your last meal. Pat yourself on the back for eating the sensible way. You will be able to maintain this for the rest of your life. You CAN be successful!

Printed in Great Britain
by Amazon

87105704R00038